An Adult Coloring Book Featuring Funny, Humorous & Stress Relieving Designs for Occupational Therapists

By © Neo coloration

Thank you for purchasing this title, we hope you enjoy coloring this book! Neo Coloration is a young start-up dedicated to creating a variety of adult coloring books.

We love what we do and everyday we do as we can to improve our products to provide you with the best coloring experience. Your feedback is important as well if you have any, don't hesitate to contact us at neocoloration@mail.com

Without your voice, we don't exist.
Please support us and leave a review!
Thank you!

Coloring can enhance individuation and promote self-discovery. Focusing on the lines of the pattern helps reduce stress and anxiety, stay present at the moment, easing anxiety about the past and worries about the future. besides getting a dose of humor and laughter that relaxes your whole body and decreases stress hormones etc...

Occupational Therapists help patients improve, regain, and develop the skills needed for day to day life and work. They also provide long-term patient care and acute patient care. They're truly superheroes in disguise!
Being an OT isn't easy and can be very stressful. Studies have shown that coloring is one of the best stress-relieving activities. Every therapist deserves a dose of humor and a moment of relaxation. Enjoy the snarky Occupational therapist's life with each page you color.

This book contains 26 pages of funny and humorous Occupational Therapist related designs and sayings surrounded By Intricate details, beautiful patterns, artworks, etc... Relax and enjoy some good vibes that will level up your confidence and will give you encouragement throughout the daily stress of life.

- Black background reverse pages to reduce bleed-through.
- Each page is single-sided for getting the best coloring experience.

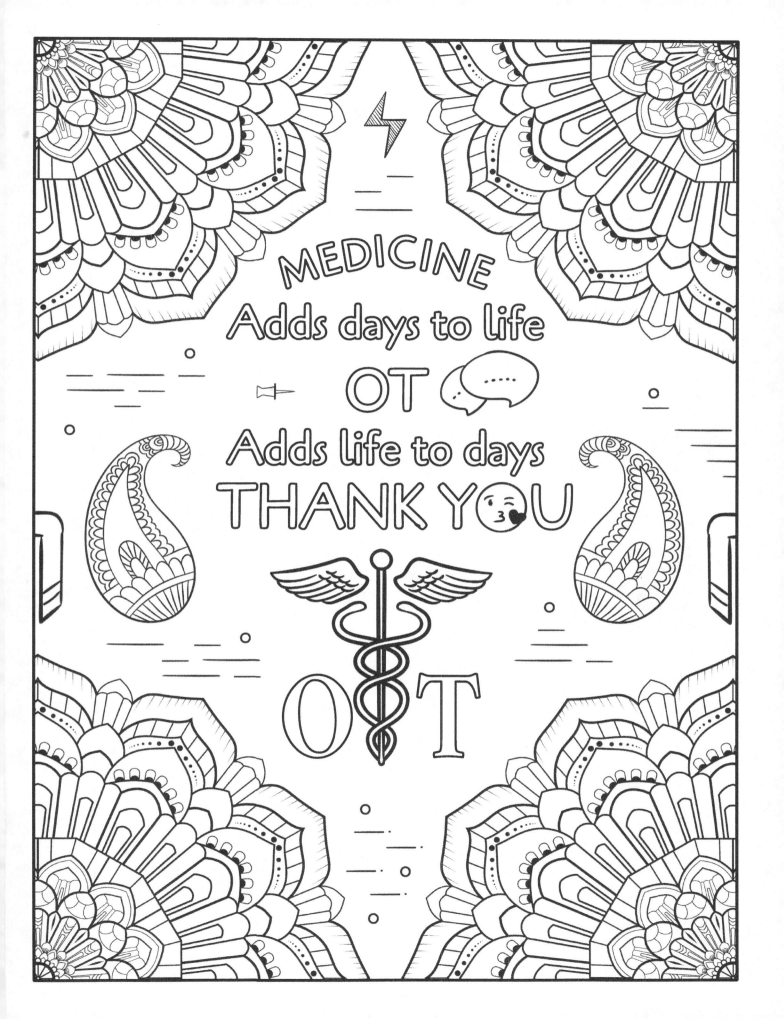

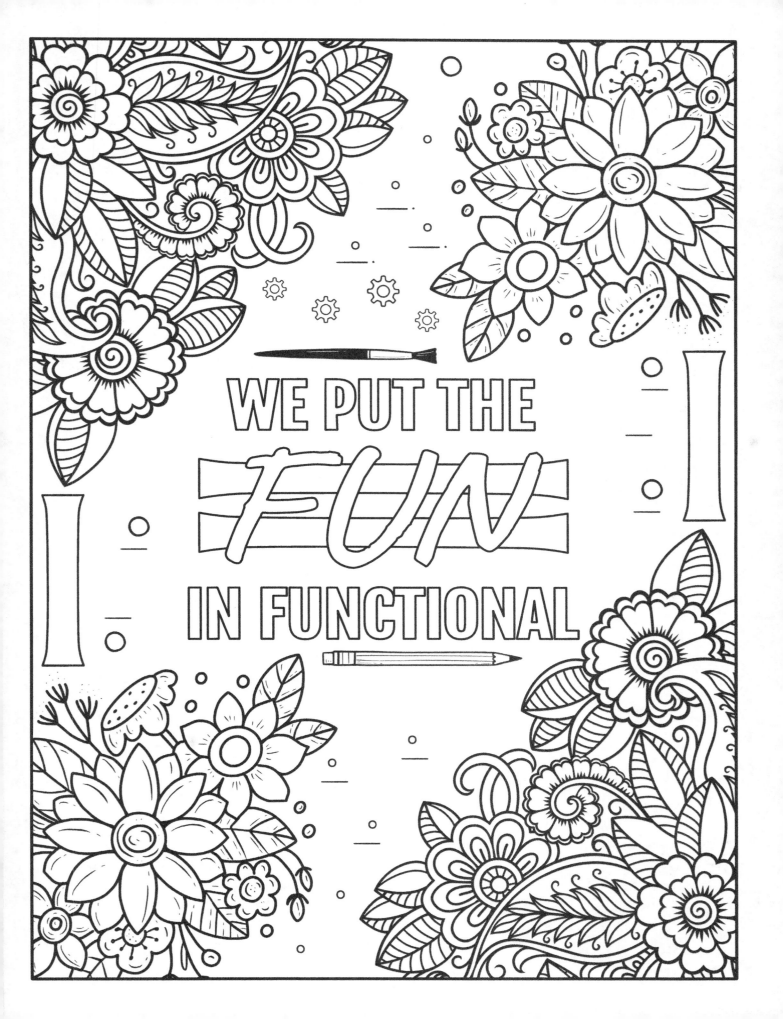

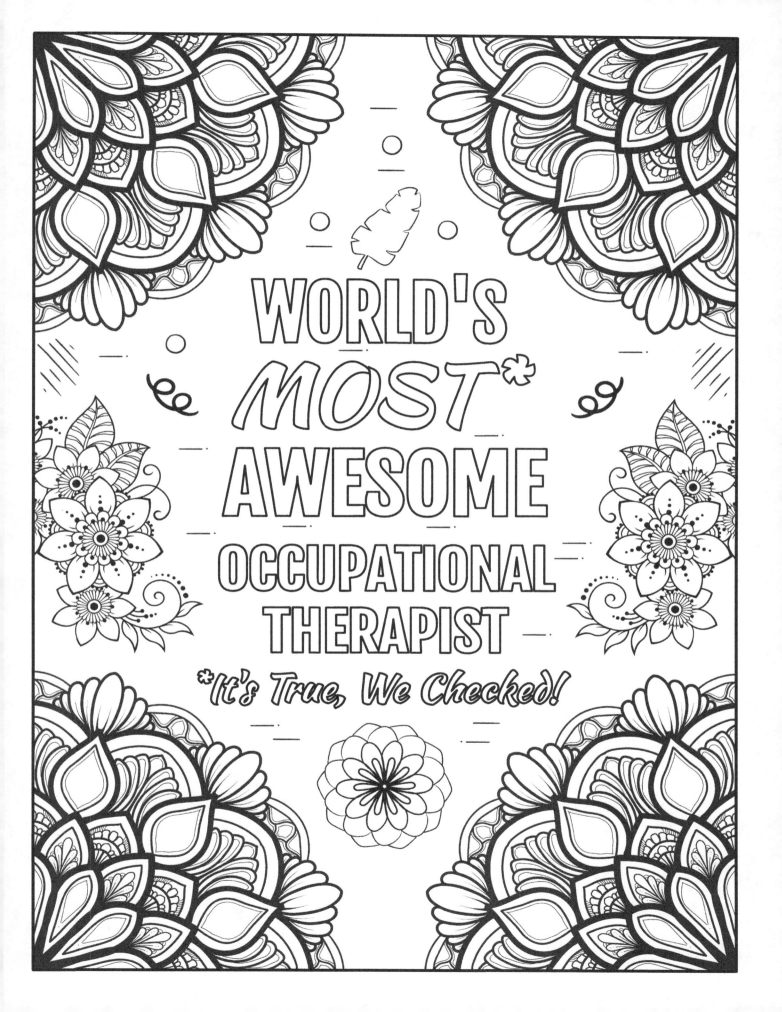

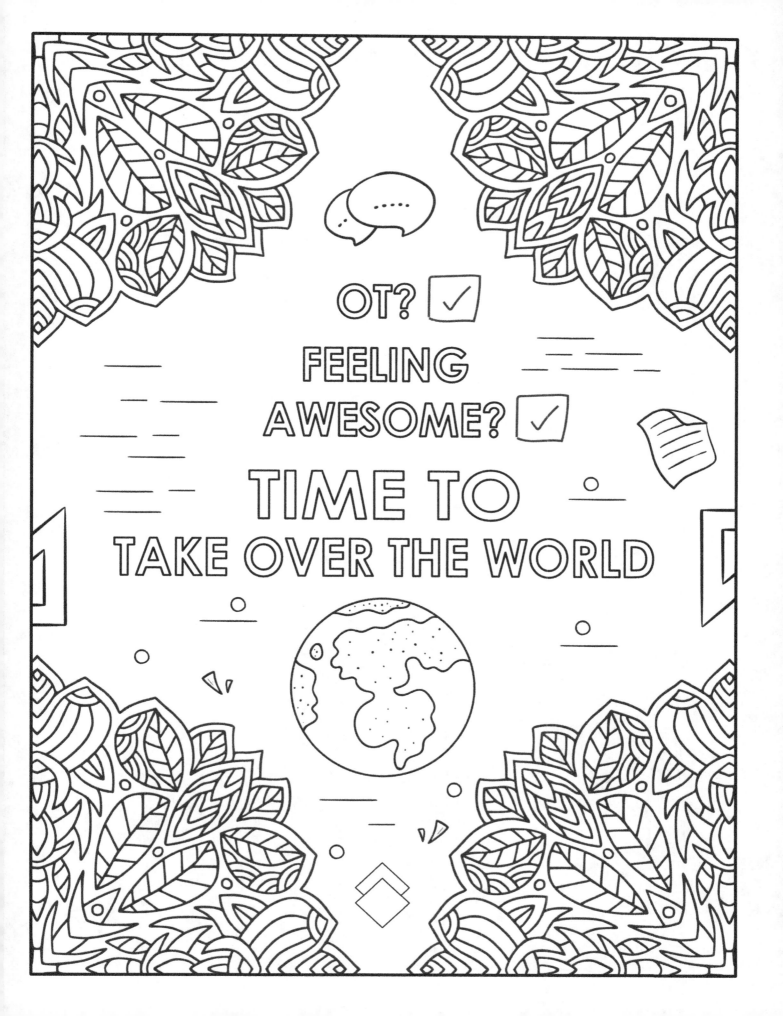

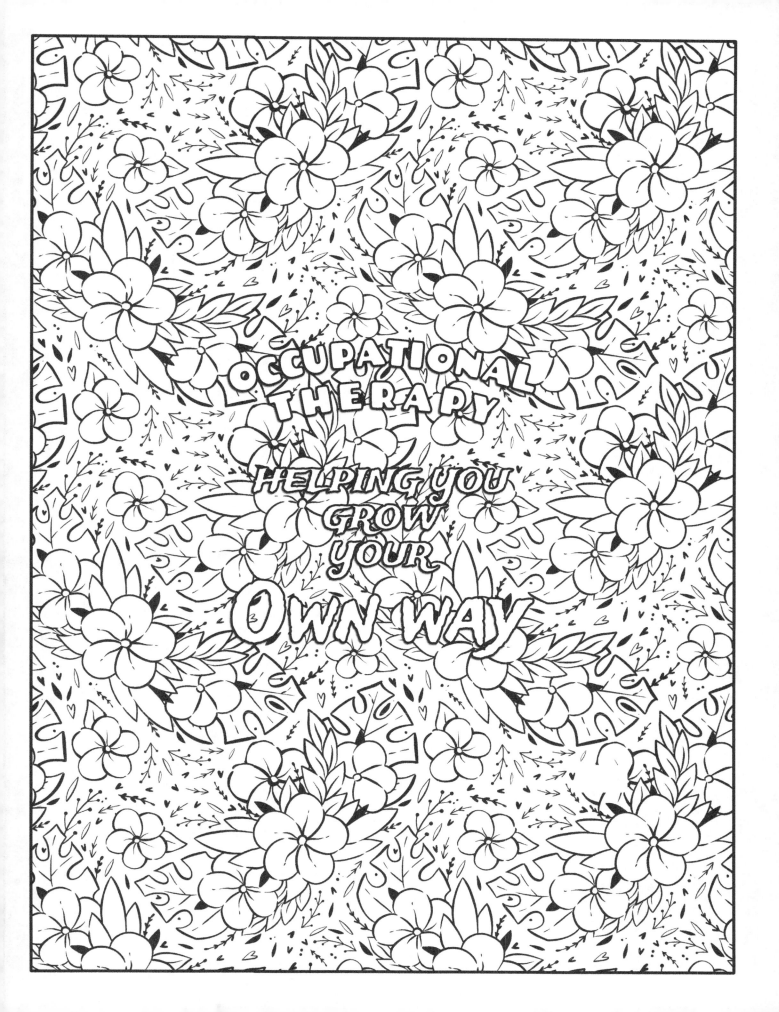

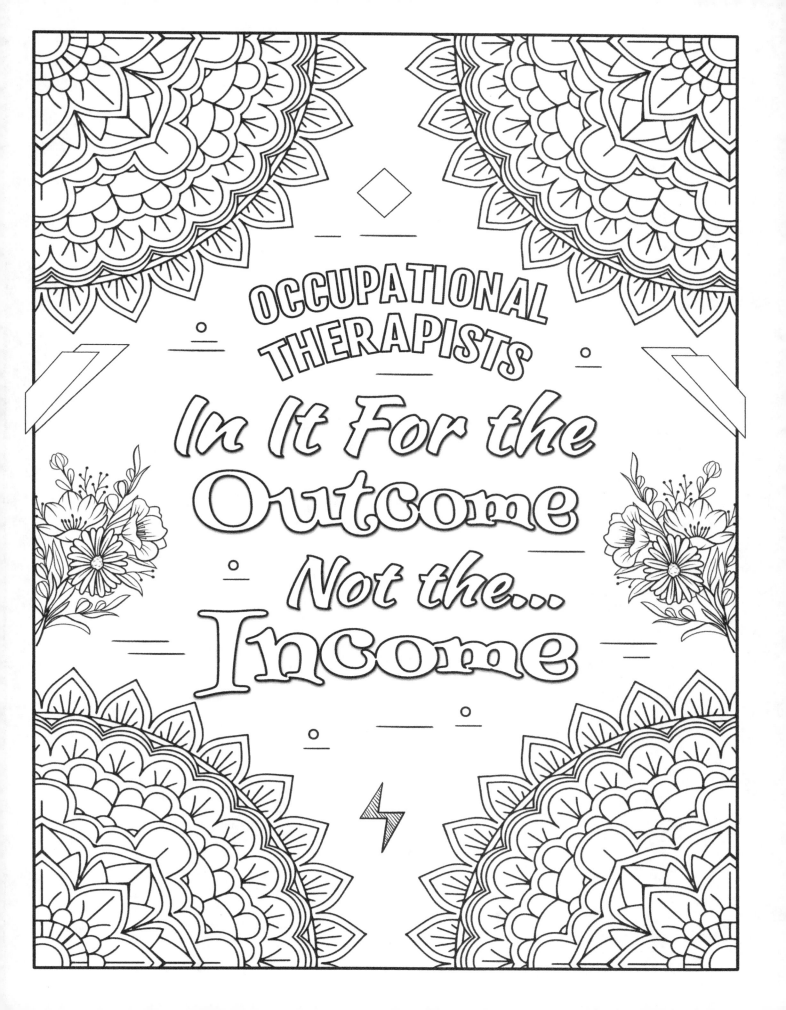

OCCUPATIONAL THERAPISTS
In It For the Outcome Not the... Income

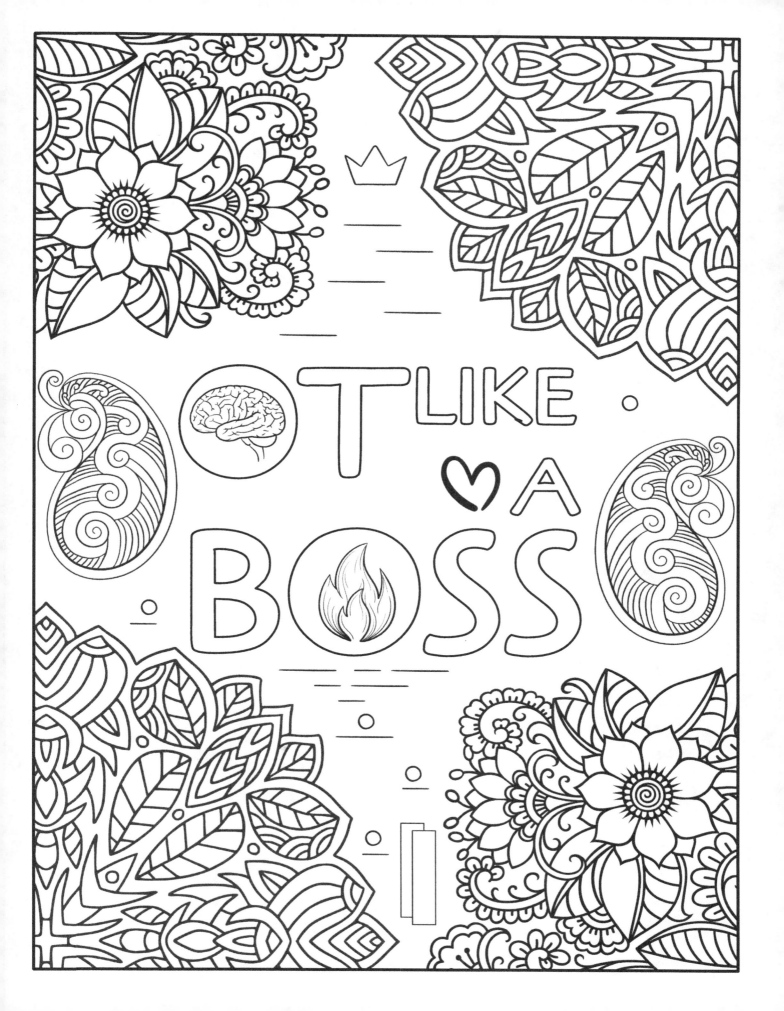

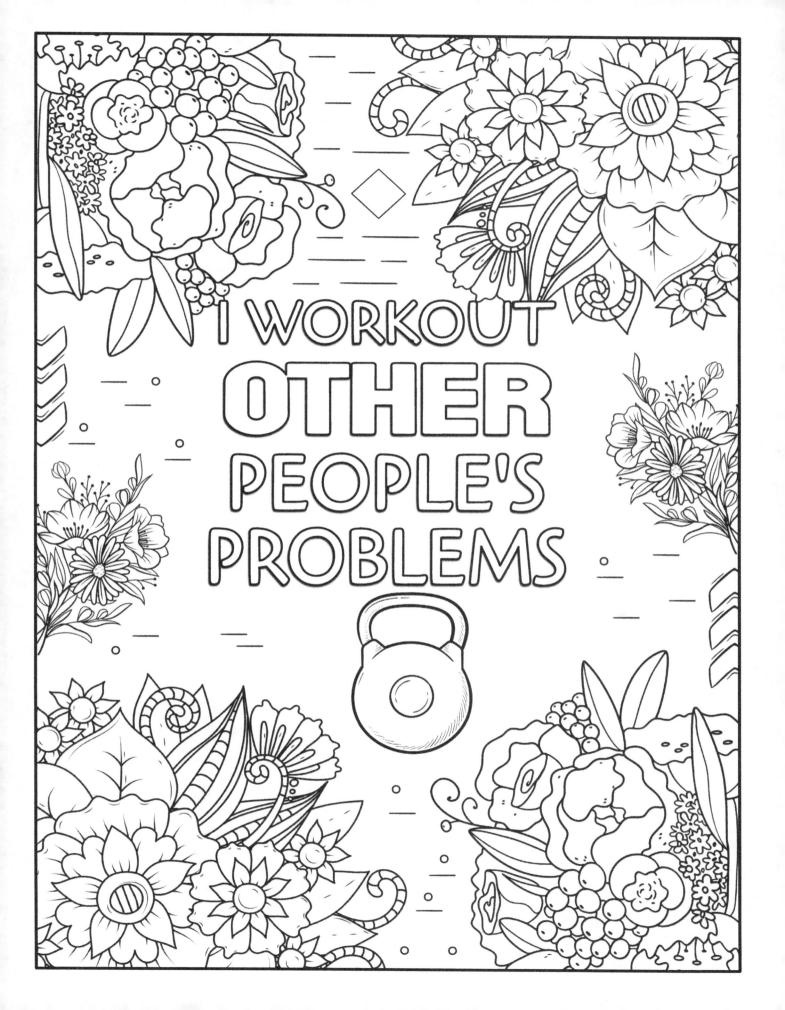

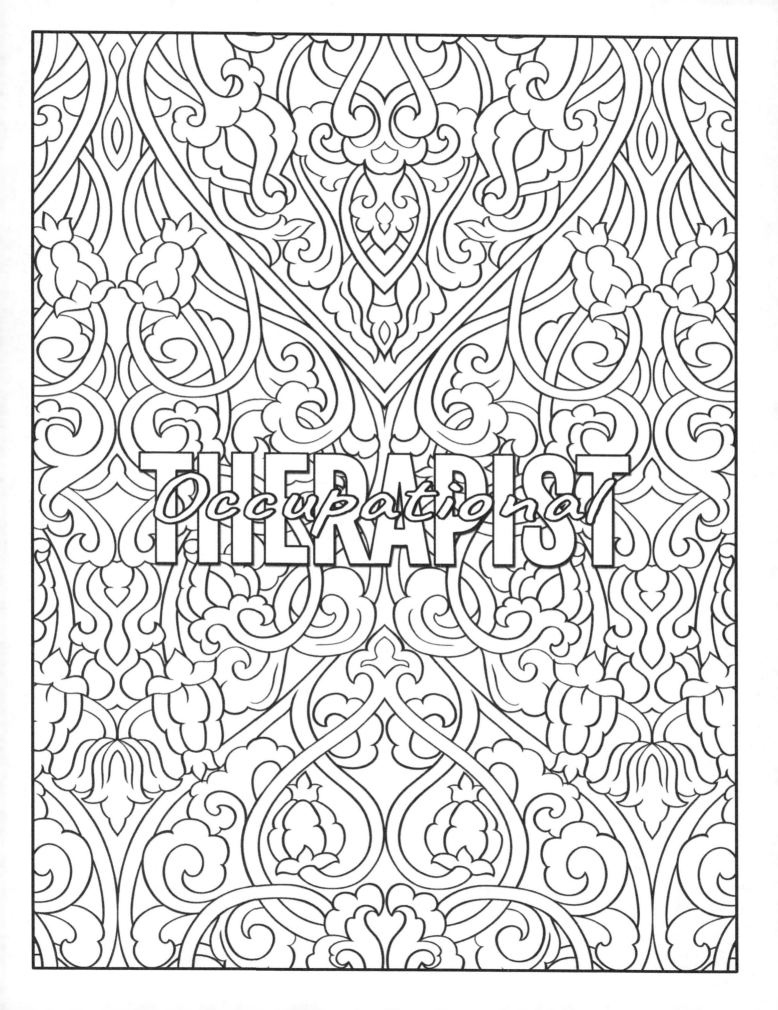

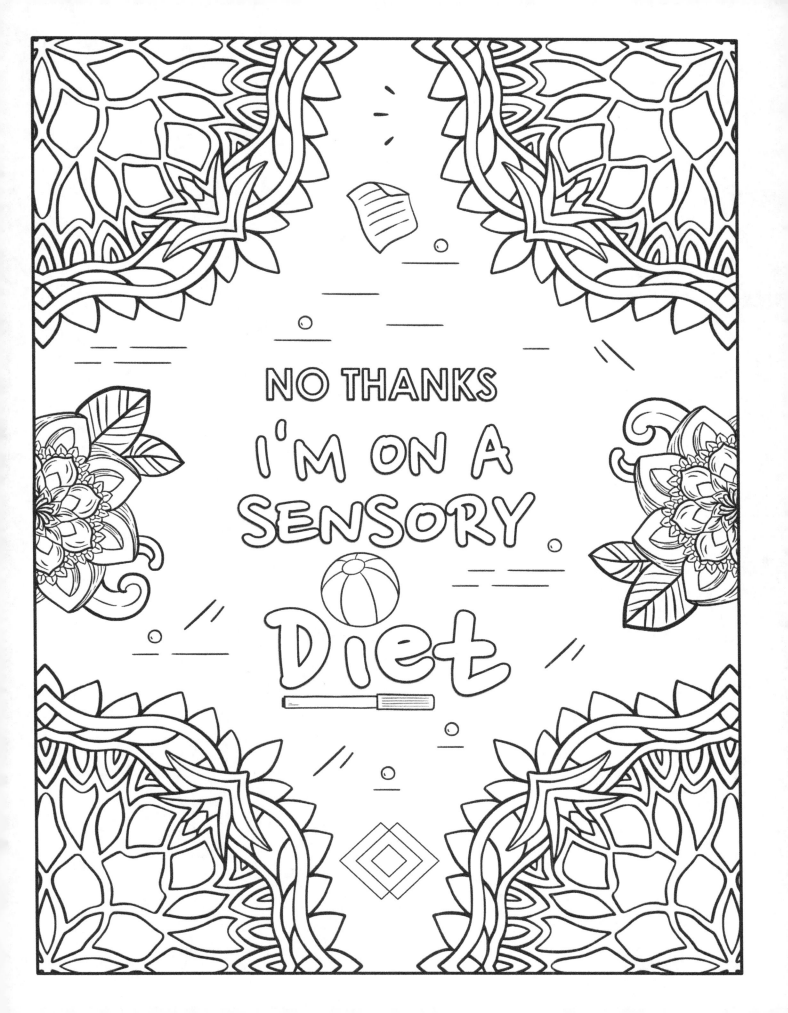

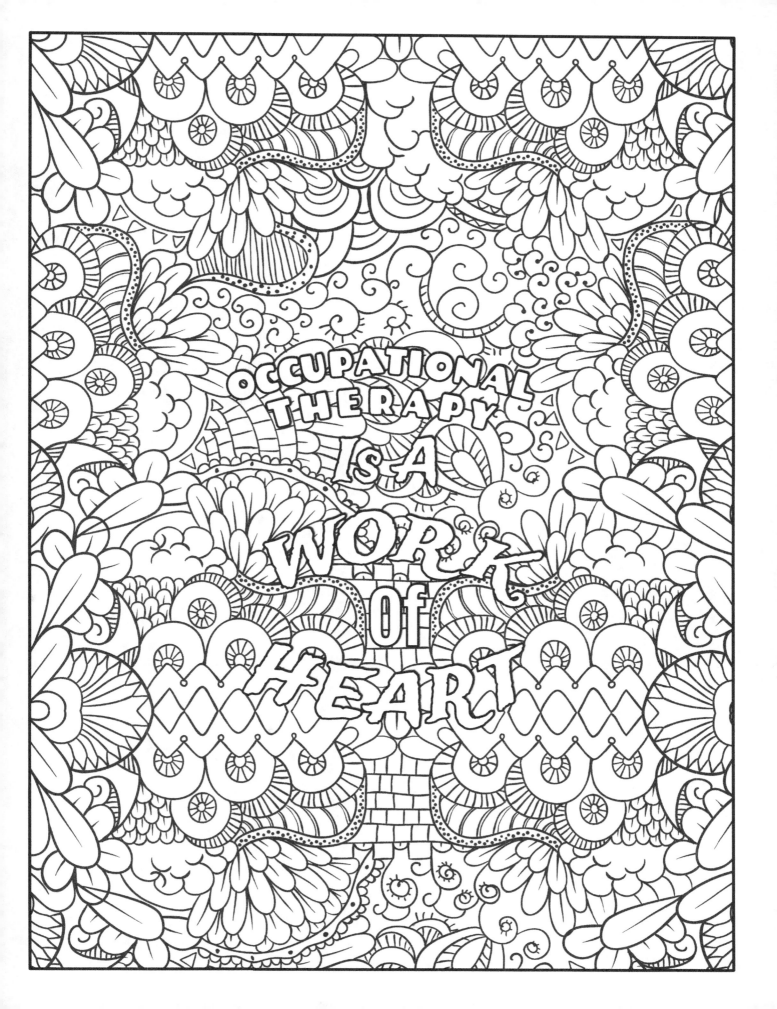

OCCUPATIONAL THERAPY IS A WORK OF HEART

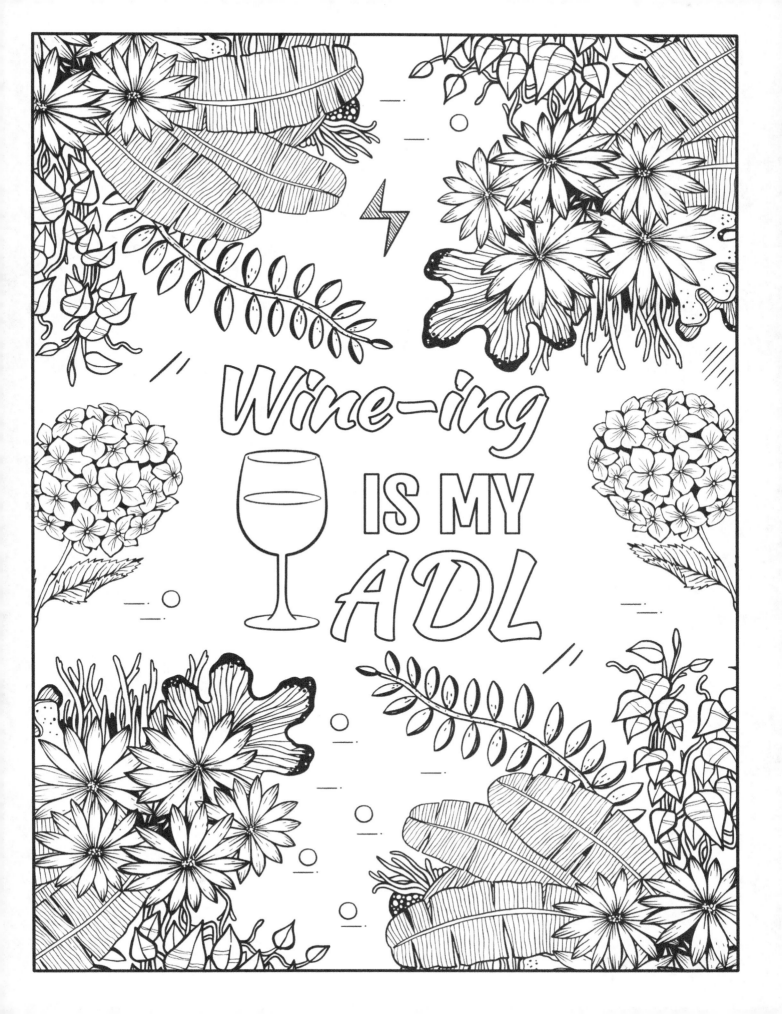

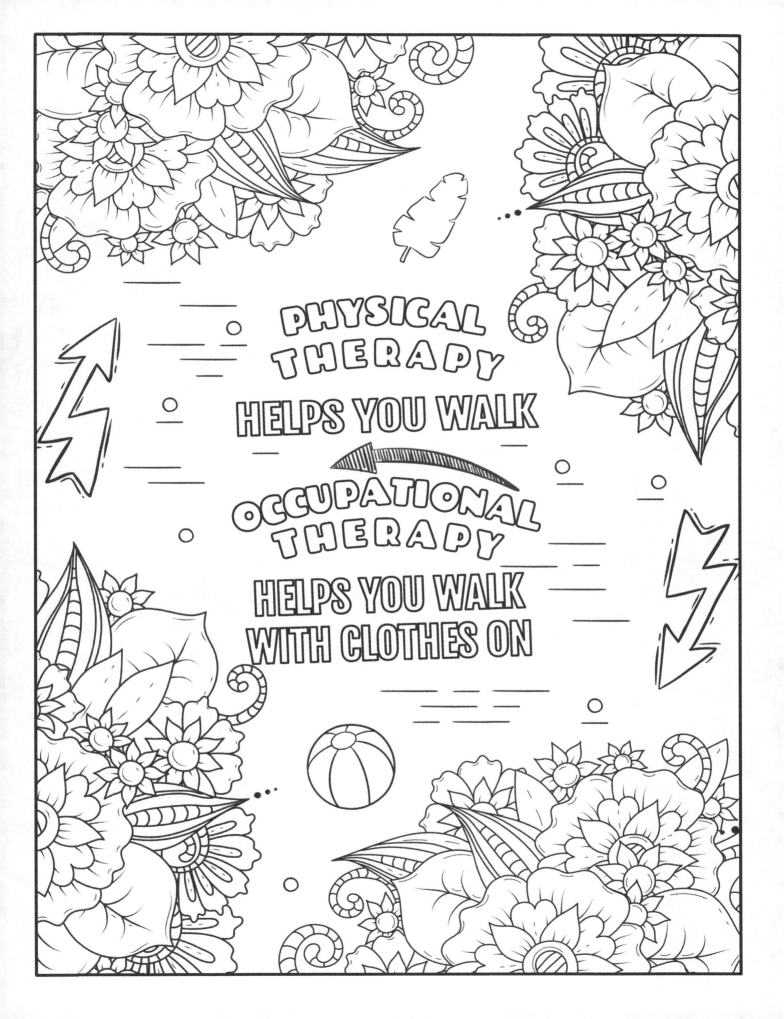

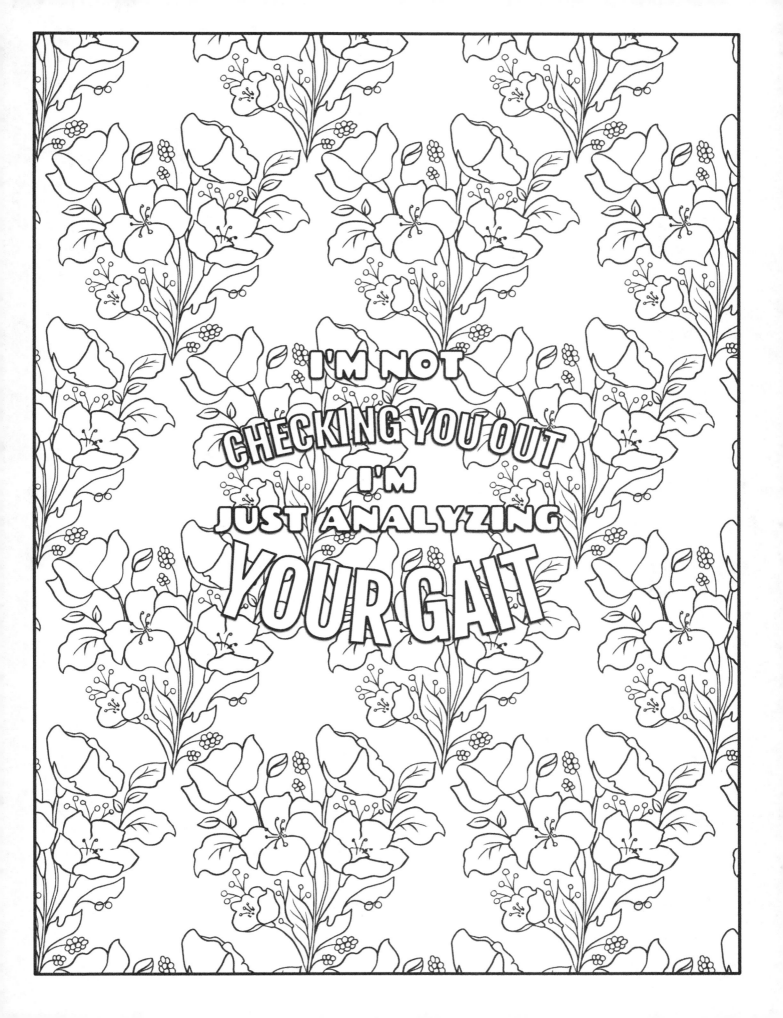

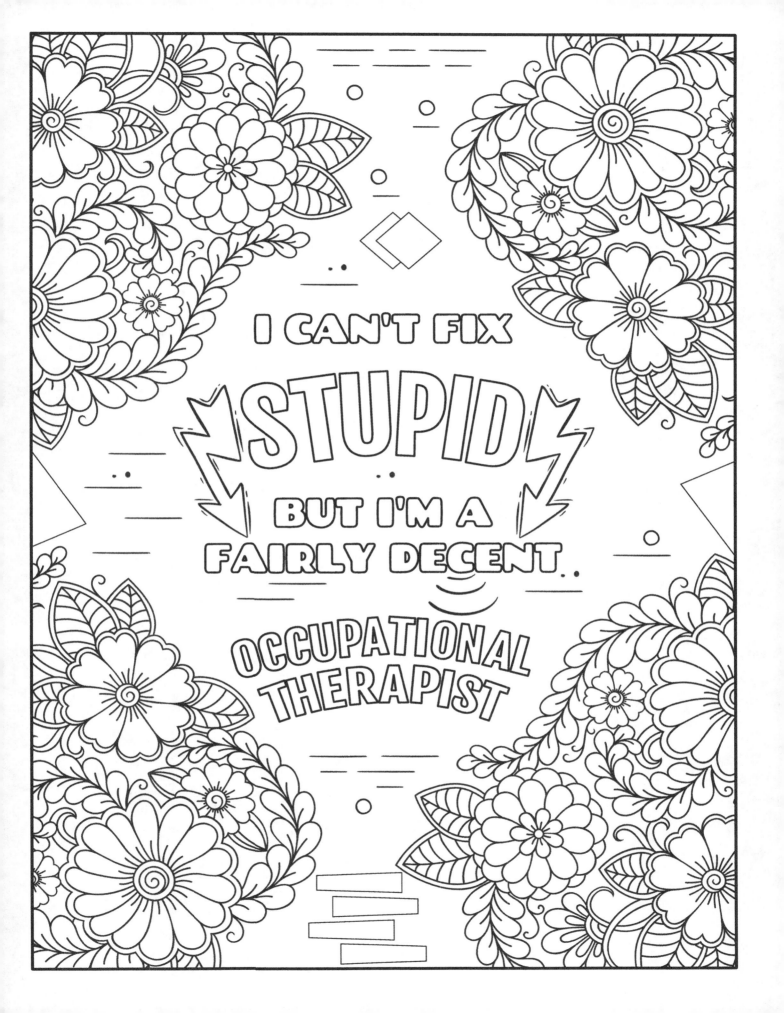

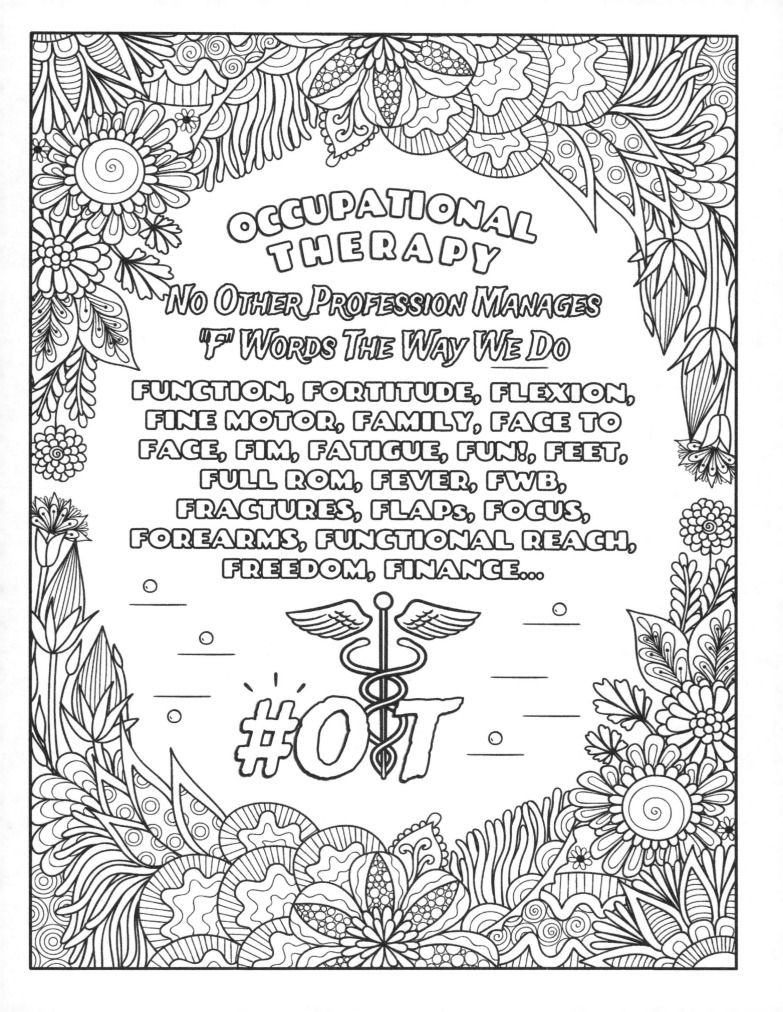

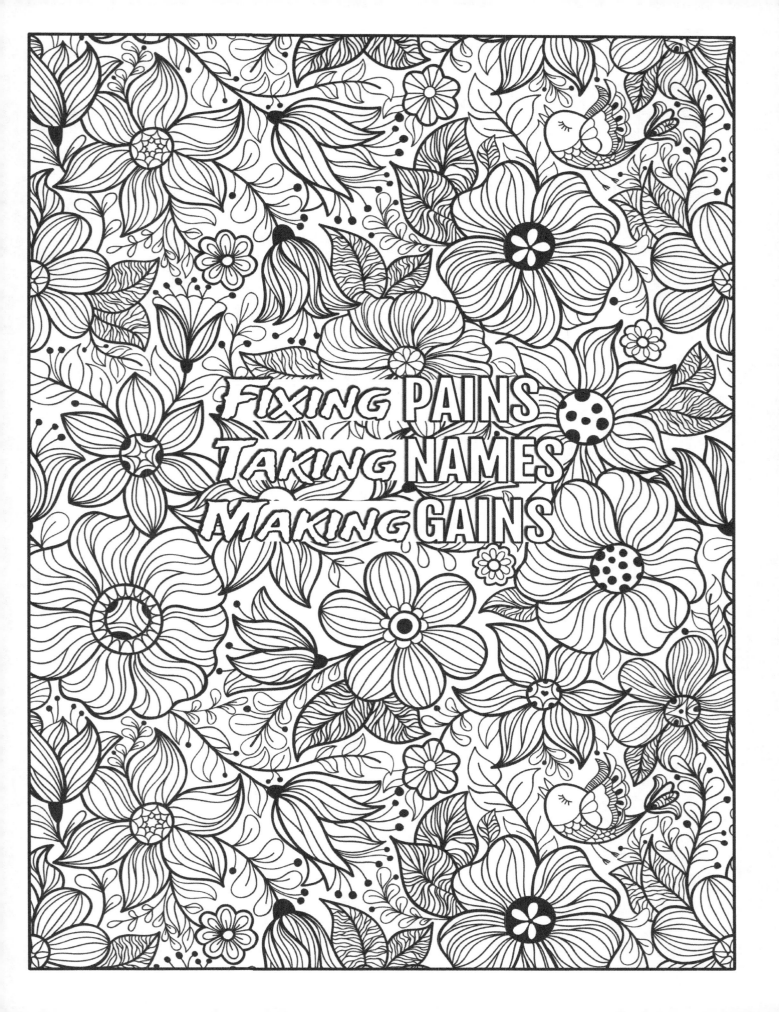

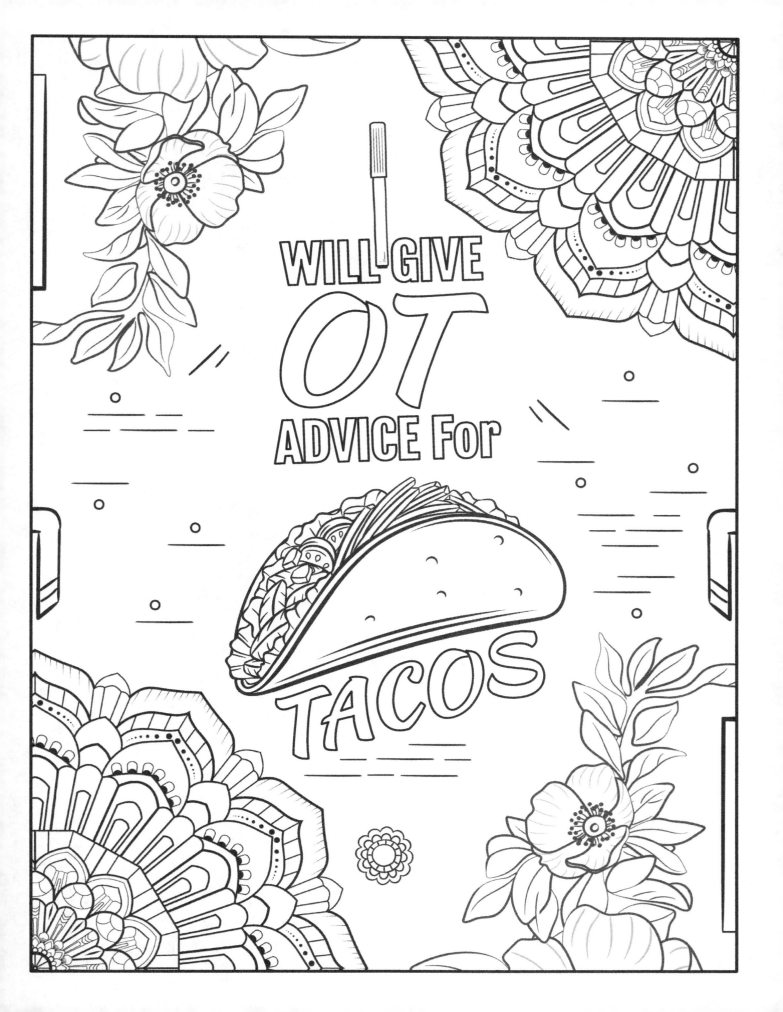

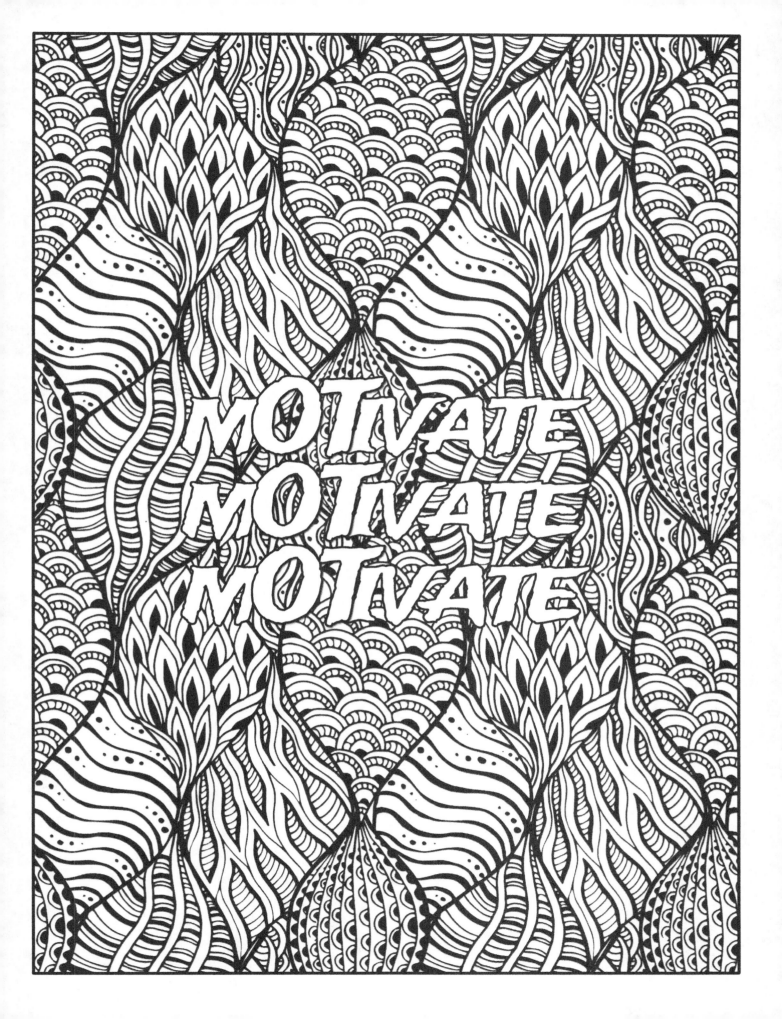

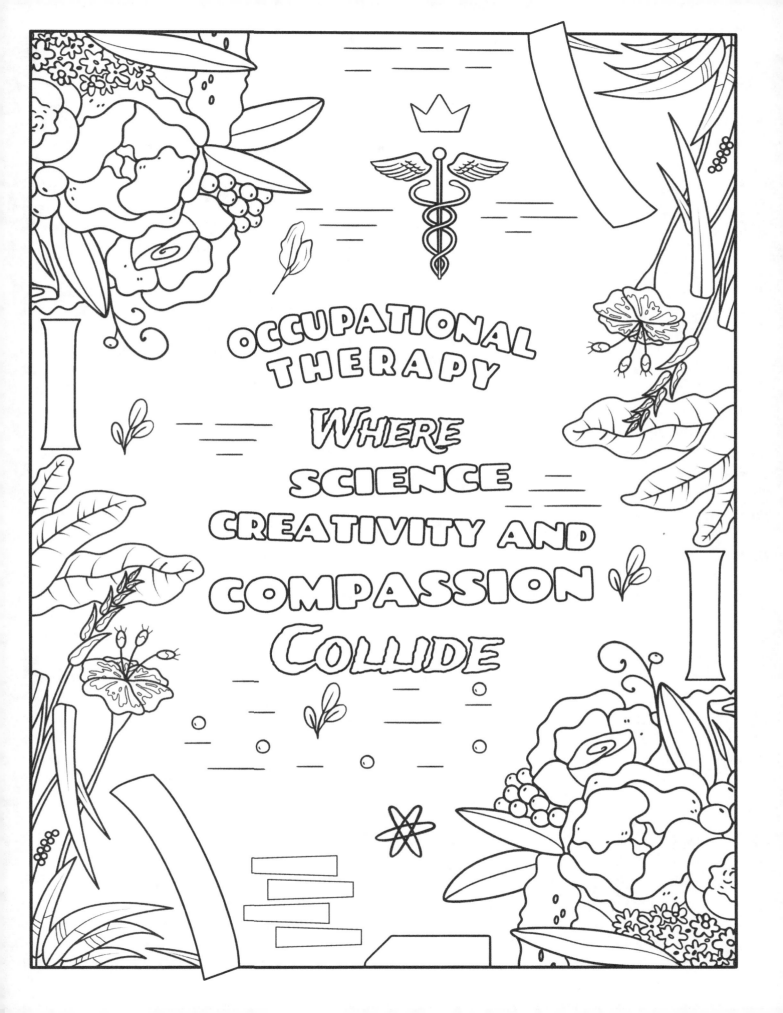

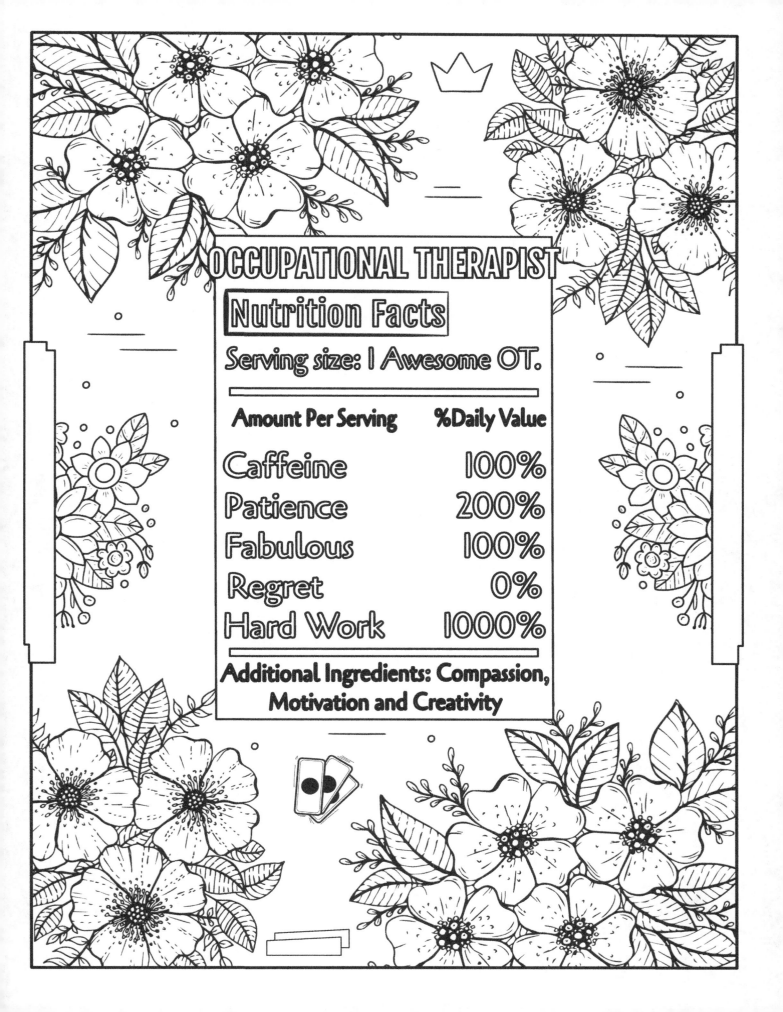

OCCUPATIONAL THERAPIST

Nutrition Facts

Serving size: 1 Awesome OT.

Amount Per Serving	%Daily Value
Caffeine	100%
Patience	200%
Fabulous	100%
Regret	0%
Hard Work	1000%

Additional Ingredients: Compassion, Motivation and Creativity

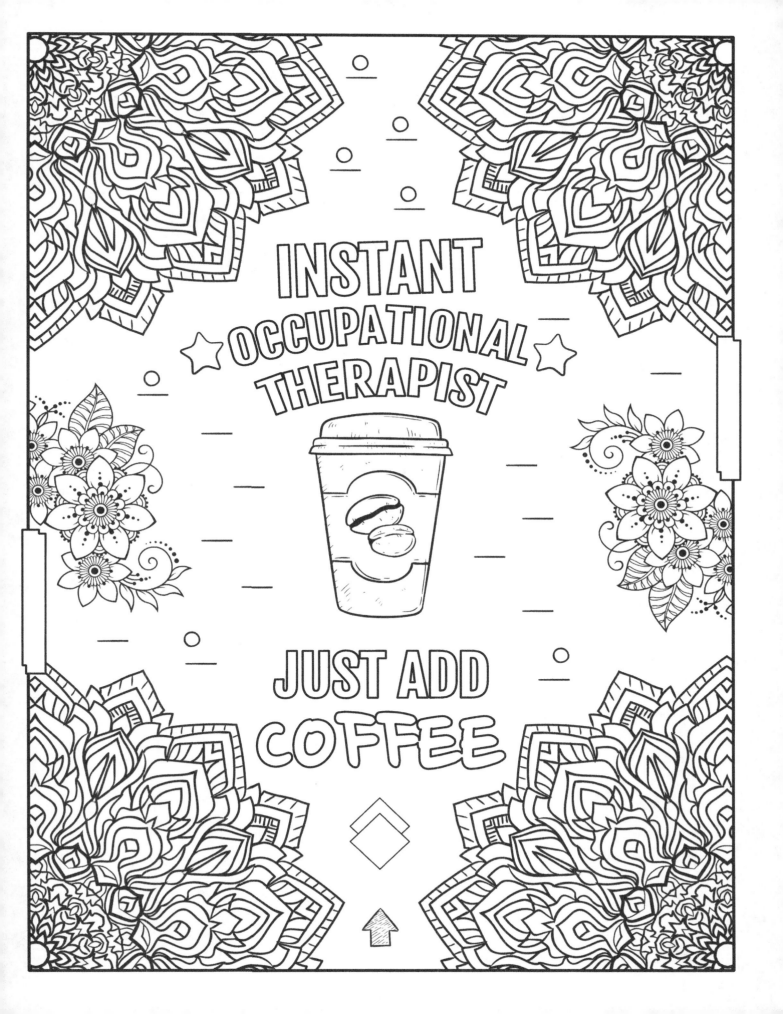

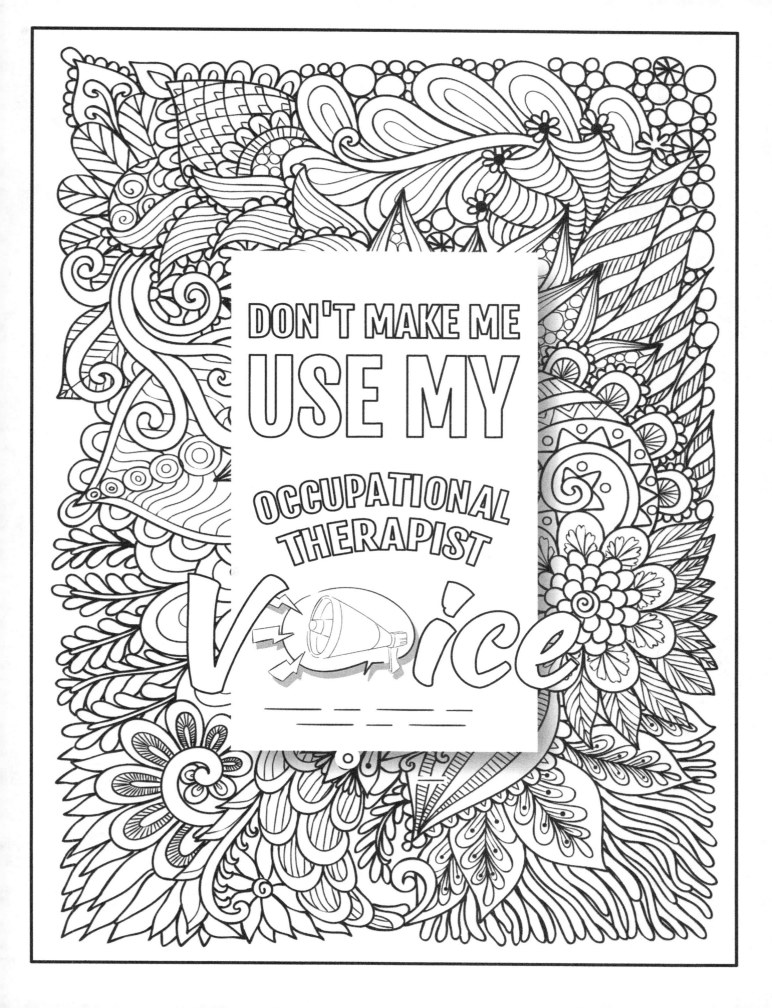

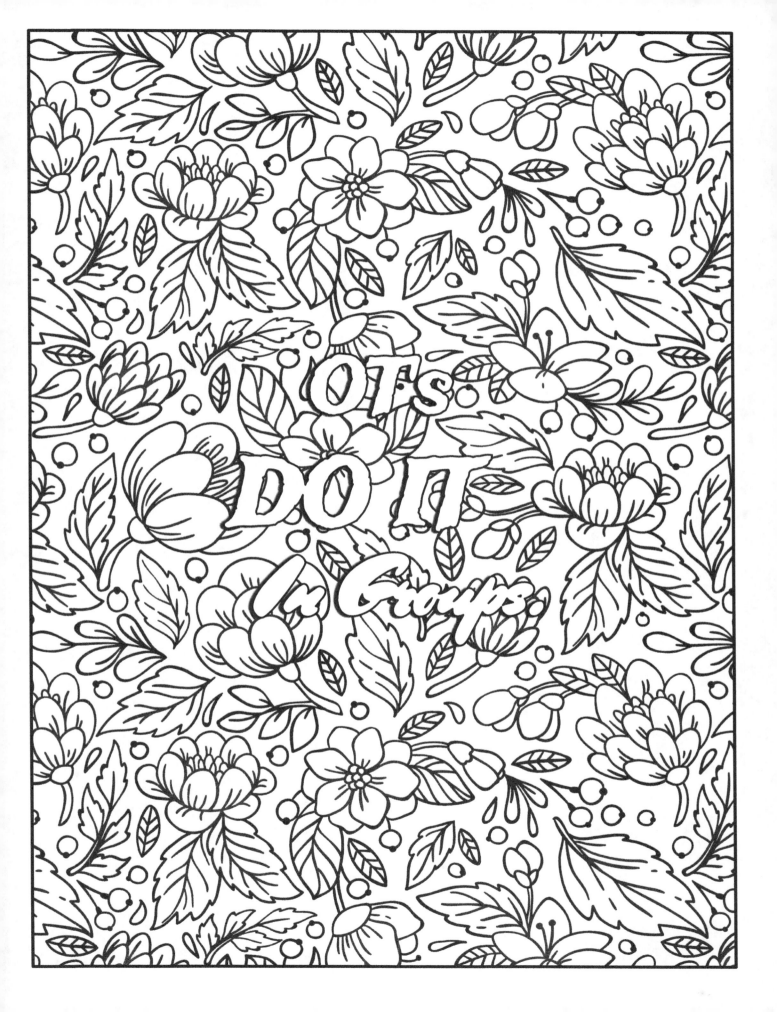

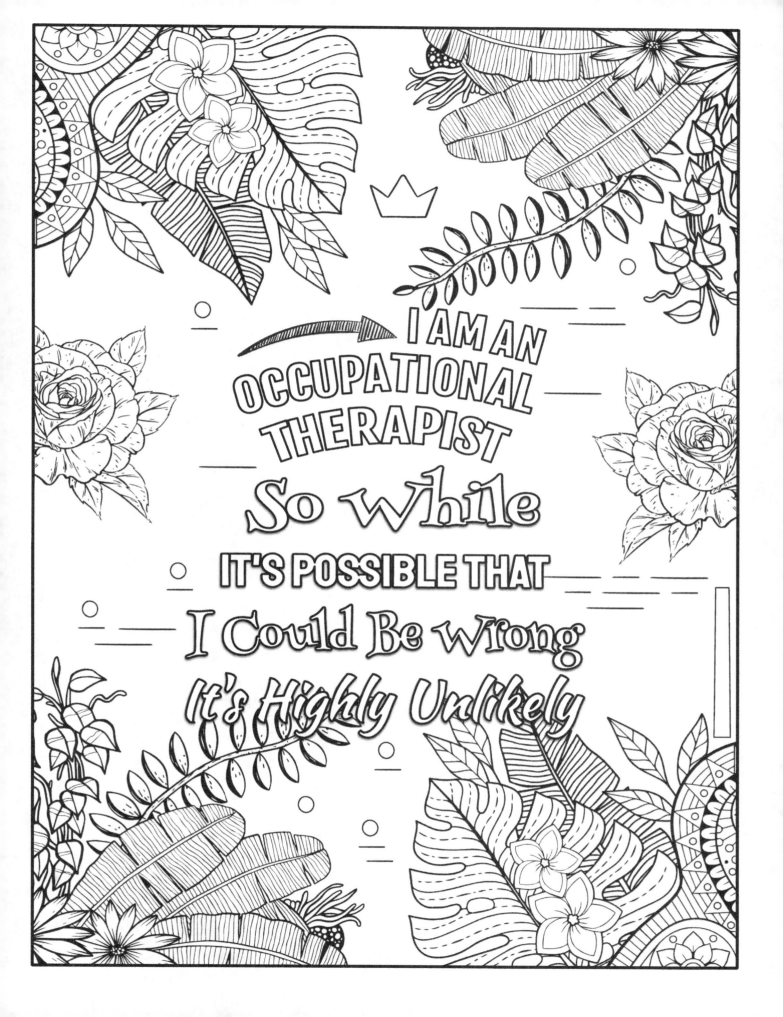

I AM AN OCCUPATIONAL THERAPIST So While IT'S POSSIBLE THAT I Could Be Wrong It's Highly Unlikely

Color test page

Color test page

Made in the USA
Middletown, DE
29 March 2024

52292801R00038